YOU AND YOUR THYROID

By the same author:

- Diet and Diabetes
- You and Your Diabetes
- Diabetes Quiz Book
- Living with Type 1 Diabetes
- मधुमेह एवं आपका भोजन
- जीवन मधुमेह के संग
- हृदय रोग और आप: रोग, उपचार एवं सावधानियाँ
- डायबिटीज प्रश्नोत्तरी

About the Author

Dr. Ashok Jhingan (birth 1949) M.B.B.S, M.D. (Medicine) is the Director of Delhi Diabetes Research Centre, New Delhi. He has been tirelessly working in the field of Diabetes and Thyroid disorders for the last forty years. He and his team are the recipient of three Guinness World records. At present, he is the Senior Director, Obesity and Metabolic Department, B.L.K-Max Hospital, New Delhi. He has also been associated as Senior Consultant, Department of Medicine, with Jaipur Golden Hospital, National Heart Institute and Primus Hospital, New Delhi.

Dr. Jhingan started his journey in a village in Morena, M.P.. After his schooling in Morena, he did his M.B.B.S. and M.D. from GRMC, Gwalior. At an early age, he was impressed by his father's dedication to community outreach in Medical Services (Father also being a doctor) and that became his life's mission.

After extensive community outreach in the field of Diabetes by organizing Health Melas and seminars for awareness of general masses, Dr. Jhingan has made significant contributions to the field of thyroid health. His work has focussed on improving the diagnosis and treatment of thyroid disorders by advancing the understanding of thyroid hormone regulations and developing innovative treatment protocols.

Dr. Jhingan's tireless and persistent efforts led to a remarkable change wherein CBSE allowed mid-exam snacks for Type 1 diabetic children in the Board examinations. Dr. Jhingan's unique concept of Peer Group Support for Type 1 diabetics and community empowerment has transformed these children into confident and successful individusls. Dr. Jhingan's You-Tube presence is commendable and his videos are widely viewed.

Dr. Jhingan has authored many books on Diabetes which have been appreciated by the Masses.

YOU AND YOUR THYROID

THE COMPLETE HANDBOOK OF MANAGING THYROID AND ITS COMPLICATIONS

Dr. Ashok Jhingan, M.D.
Director, Delhi Diabetes Research Centre, New Delhi
Senior Director, BLK-Max Diabetes,
Obesity & Metabolic Centre

GOLDEN JUBILEE Concept 50 YEARS 1974-2024

CONCEPT PUBLISHING COMPANY PVT. LTD.
NEW DELHI - 110 059

ISBN: 978-93-6344-275-7

First Published 2025

Published and Printed by

Concept Since 1974

Concept Publishing Company Pvt. Ltd.
A/15-16, Commercial Block, Mohan Garden
New Delhi-110059 (India)
T: +91-11-41101460
E: publishing@conceptpub.com, *W*: www.conceptpub.com

Cataloging in Publication--Courtesy: D.K. Agencies (P) Ltd. <docinfo@dkagencies.com>

Jhiṅgana, E. Ke. (Aśoka Ke.), 1949- **author.**
You and your thyroid : the complete handbook of managing thyroid and its complications/ Dr. Ashok Jhingan, M.D.
pages cm
ISBN 9789363442757

1. Thyroid gland--Diseases--Handbooks, manuals, etc. I. Title.

LCC RC655.J56 2025 | DDC 616.44 23

In memory of
my parents who taught me the value of perseverance, sincerity, truthfulness, compassion, gratitude and empathy that I follow till today.

Foreword

In this comprehensive guide to thyroid health, we dive deep into the often-misunderstood world of Thyroid gland. This book is designed to empower readers with knowledge about the thyroid, a small but powerful gland that significantly impacts our overall health and well-being. Covering a wide range of topics, from the basics of thyroid anatomy and function to the complexities of thyroid disorders such as hypothyroidism, hyperthyroidism, and autoimmune conditions like Hashimoto's thyroiditis and Graves' disease, this book provides valuable insights for anyone looking to understand more about their thyroid health.

Through a combination of patients experiences and the latest research, we shed light on the often-overlooked symptoms of thyroid dysfunction—like fatigue, weight changes, depression, and anxiety—and explain the diagnostic tests and criteria used by healthcare professionals. The book provides clear, actionable guidance on navigating various treatment options, from conventional approaches such as medication and surgery to alternative therapies, including diet, exercise, and stress management techniques that support thyroid health.

This book is not just about managing thyroid conditions; it's about empowering individuals to reclaim their health, improve their quality of life, and achieve lasting well-being.

With a focus on patient empowerment, this book aims to improve your thyroid health, offering clear explanations and actionable steps to help readers take control of their health journey. Whether you are newly diagnosed or have been managing thyroid issues for years, or are simply looking to understand more about this essential gland, "You and your Thyroid" is an invaluable resource on your path to wellness.

Prof. Dr. Vinod Kumar M.D.
Physician, Geriatrician & Endocrinologist
Patron, Indian Academy of Geriatrics
Formerly: Professor of Medicine, AIIMS, Delhi

Author's Note

In today's fast-paced world, the health of our thyroid gland often goes unnoticed until its dysfunction significantly impacts our lives. The thyroid, though small in size, plays an immense role in regulating our metabolism, energy levels, and overall well-being. When thyroid disorders arise, they can lead to a myriad of symptoms that affect not only our physical health but also our mental and emotional states.

As a dedicated expert in the field, I have spent years studying the intricacies of the thyroid gland and its profound effect on the human body.

One of the greatest strengths of this book is its ability to explain complex medical concepts, making them accessible to everyone. Whether you are a patient, caregiver, or healthcare professional, you will find the information presented in these pages to be both enlightening and actionable. I skillfully break down the types of thyroid disorders, their symptoms, diagnostic methods, and treatment options, providing a holistic approach to thyroid health.

Beyond the medical explanations, this book also emphasises the importance of a balanced lifestyle in managing thyroid conditions. This book offers insights into nutrition, exercise, stress management, and other lifestyle factors that play a crucial role in supporting thyroid function. By integrating these practical tips into daily life, readers can take proactive steps towards better health and improved quality of life.

As you embark on this journey through the world of thyroid health, I encourage you to absorb the wealth of knowledge and wisdom. Let this book be your guide to understanding your thyroid and achieving a balanced and vibrant life.

Dr. Ashok Jhingan

Acknowledgements

There are so many people that I would like to thank since I was never alone in this journey and this book wouldn't have been possible if it weren't for the support of many people, so understandably, the list gets longer.

I owe more than that I can describe to my late parents Dr. R.N. Jhingan, my father and my mother, Savitri Jhingan, who taught me the value of perseverance, sincerity, truthfulness, compassion, gratitude and empathy that I follow till now.

My wife Dr. Kamalesh Jhingan who has always been my pillar of strength and has given valuable support and has also been the proof reader of this book. I couldn't have done without her help and encouragement.

My children and my grandchildren, I thank you all for your unconditional love and support.

I thank my team, clinical and para medical staff at Delhi Diabetes Research Centre—Dr. Padam Sharma, Sr. Dietician Preeti Bajaj, Saji Thomas, Ritika, Nitish for their valuable support.

I extend my heartfelt thanks to my patients, whose experiences and personal stories have been a constant source of inspiration. Your courage and resilience has driven me to dive deeper into understanding thyroid health and advocate for better care.

I am grateful to my teachers and professors at GRMC, Gwalior for guiding me in my career.

I am profoundly grateful to my colleagues and mentors in the medical field. Your insights, advice and encouragement has been invaluable in shaping the contents of this book.

Finally, to my readers, thank you for your interest in this book. I hope the information and guidance provided here will empower you to take charge of your thyroid health and lead a healthier and more fulfilling life.

With sincere gratitude,

Dr. Ashok Jhingan

Contents

Introduction

Thyroid gland is a small butterfly shaped gland, located at the front of your neck under the skin. It is an important gland which controls many of the important bodily functions by producing and releasing thyroid hormone like Thyroxin (T4) and Triiodothyronine (T3).

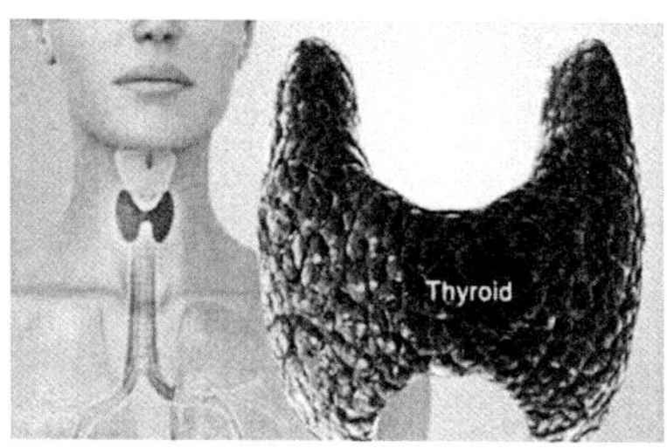

Function of the Thyroid gland is to control metabolism. By this process, body transforms the food we consume into energy. All the cells in the body needs energy to function.This hormone plays a key role in regulating blood pressure, body temperature, heart rate, metabolism and the reaction of the body to other hormones. Thyroid gland not only controls metabolic processes, but also the activation response of body to other hormones.

What happens if thyroid does not function properly?

Thyroid problems start when thyroid gland produces either too much or too little of the hormones.

This leads to

- **Goiter*:** An enlargement of the thyroid gland.
- **Hypothyroidism:** When thyroid gland does not make enough thyroid hormones (underactive).
- **Hyperthyroidism:** When thyroid gland makes more thyroid hormones than body needs (overactive).
- **Thyroid cancer.**
- **Thyroiditis**: Swelling and inflammation of the thyroid gland.
- **Thyroid nodules:** Lumps in the thyroid gland.

What are the symptoms of Thyroid Disease?

- Unintentional weight gain or weight loss.
- Feeling hungry more often.
- Faster or irregular heart rate (as well as palpitations of the heart).
- Trembling of the hands (inability to keep them steady).
- Being more susceptible to heat as well as sweating more easily.
- Changes in periods, bowel movements, sleep cycle, fatigue.
- Changes in skin, hair and nails (thinning, becoming more brittle).

Disorder of the thyroid gland

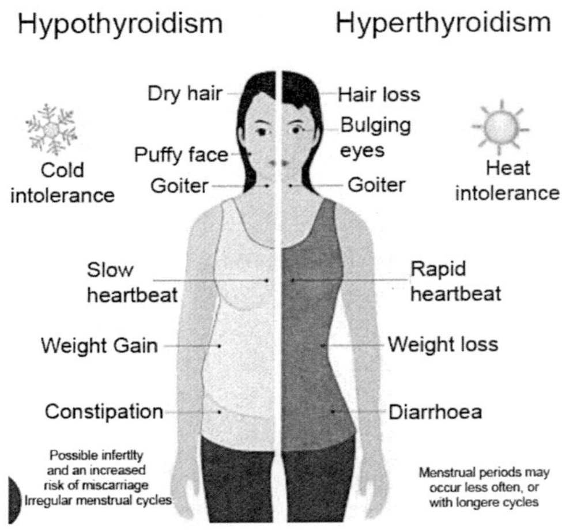

- Swelling at the base of the neck.

What are the tests done for thyroid problems?

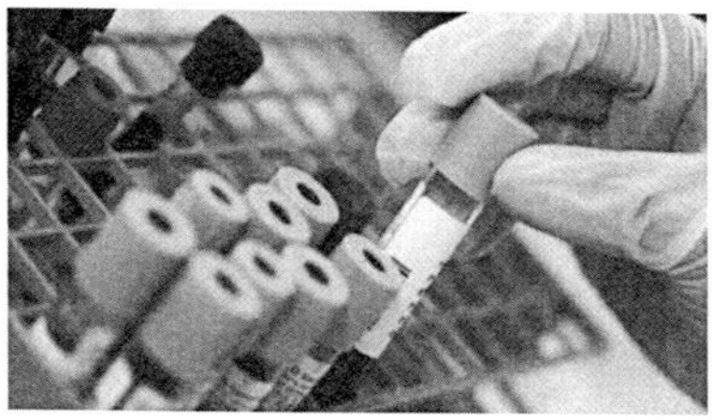

Thyroid Stimulating Hormone (TSH) is a hormone secreted by the pituitary gland that tells the thyroid gland how much T3 and T4 to make. Estimation of serum TSH is a simple blood test which is done fasting but does not require fasting if you take Thyroid medicine then this test is done about 4-5 hours after taking the medicine. I would like to caution you to avoid Biotin supplements (present in many hair and nail supplements) for about one week before the test as Biotin can interfere with laboratory test.

Generally, TSH varies between 0.5 to 4.50 mIU/L, however, laboratory specific reference/ranges should be used. Also the upper limit may not be same for specific population's example for elderly we liberalize the TSH target up to 7-8. At the age of 65 TSH value of 7 is considered normal and at 75 years TSH value of 8 is normal.

High TSH usually means you have **hypothyroidism (low thyroid function)**.This means your thyroid gland is not making enough hormone.Therefore, Pituitary gland increases the release of TSH (Thyroid stimulating hormone) in the blood.

A low TSH means hyperthyroidism, that means thyroid gland making too much hormone so the Pituitary glands stops making and releasing TSH (suppressed TSH).

T4

A High blood level of T4 means you have overactive thyroid or hyperthyroidism and low level means hypothyroidism.

If you are pregnant or taking oral contraceptive your T4 levels may be high.

T3

If the person is having hyperthyroidism then you may have both T4 and T3 levels on the higher side.

Thyroid Antibodies

Thyroid peroxidase antibodies (T.P.O.) are Thyroid specific antibodies and represent autoimmune Thyroid Disease. TPO antibodies are seen generally in Hashimoto's Thyroiditis. TSI Antibodies or thyroid receptors antibodies (TRAB) are specific for Graves' disease.

Levels of thyroid antibodies represent autoimmune disorders like Graves' disease, the most common cause of hyperthyroidism and Hashimoto's disease, the most common cause of hypothyroidism.

What are other tests for thyroid disorder?

- **Ultrasound of neck for thyroid:** Ultrasound is most often used to look for thyroid nodules. Ultrasound of thyroid can also reveal if the nodules have benign or suspicious appearance.
- **Thyroid scan:** This test is done to find out the shape and size of thyroid gland. This test is done by using a small amount of Radioactive iodine. One has to stop Iodine containing medicines a week before this test.
  This test helps to find out the nature of nodule, causing hyperthyroidism.
- **F.N.A.C. or Biopsy of nodule:** Ultrasound guided needle biopsy of nodule is done and a small amount of tissue is sent to the lab for finding out the nature of cells.

When and who should get the screening for thyroid?

For people without any symptoms it's recommended:

- For women of reproductive age group or desiring pregnancy establish baseline TSH, free-T4 and TPO levels and screen also during the first month of pregnancy.

- Those people who are on certain medicines, like Amiodarone/ Lithium as these medicines alter Thyroid hormone levels.
- Those patients who are on immunotherapy for cancer treatment.
- In Geriatric or elderly patients also, the thyroid screening should be done to assess the levels as many of them don't have typical symptoms. Screening at least once a year is generally recommended.

Hypothyroidism

What is hypothyroidism?

Hypothyroidism is due to insufficient thyroid hormone. Thyroid does not make enough thyroid hormone.This is also called as under-active thyroid.

What are the symptoms of hypothyroidism?

- Feeling tired.
- Gaining weight.
- Delayed periods and occasionally heavy and frequent menstrual periods.
- Constipation.
- Dry and coarse skin.
- Numbness in fingers.
- Excessive Hair fall.
- Decreased sexual interest.
- Puffiness on the eyes and face.
- Forgetfulness.
- Feeling depressed.

Hypothyroidism occurs

- When there is thyroiditis (inflammation).
- After thyroid surgery.

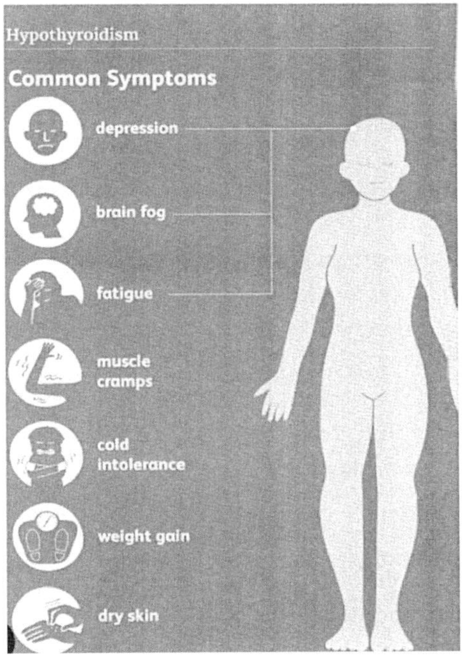

- After radioactive iodine treatment.
- Medicines like Lithium and Amiodarone.
- After radiation treatment of thyroid.
- Severe iodine deficiency.

Hypothyroidism in children

- Hypothyroidism in children can cause poor growth which leads to short stature (height).
- Delayed dental development.
- Delayed puberty.
- Poor mental growth.

How to manage hypothyroidism?

Treatment for hypothyroidism usually includes taking the thyroid hormone replacement daily, which is available as Levothyroxine Tablet.

- This medicine is taken by mouth orally in early morning other medicine like antacids or breakfast should be taken 50 minutes after this medicine. Patient starts feeling better after 2 weeks of treatment.

These medicines likely will be lifelong. Dosage may change as per the TSH levels. TSH test may be repeated after 6 to 8 weeks after taking the medicines. Too much dose of these medicines can cause tiredness, increased appetite, sleep problems, palpitations and shakiness.Therefore, regular monitoring and dose adjustment is mandatory.

Don't stop or skip taking thyroid medicines otherwise symptoms of hypothyroidism will reappear. If you miss a dose, in morning then you may take it as soon as you remember that day or take 2 tablets the next day.

Diet in hypothyroidism

- **Maintain Good intake of iodine rich foods such as eggs, milk, seafood. Use iodized salt.**
- **Avoid Soya in excess.**
- **Avoid excessive intake of cruciferous vegetables** (goitrogens) like cabbage, cauliflower and broccoli.
- **Gluten (wheat):** Gluten can also trigger thyroid inflammatory responses (AUTOIMMUNE).
- **But I don't feel this is necessary and moderate intake should be OK.**

Complications

Several complications can occur if you have an underactive thyroid that is not treated.

Heart problems

If you have an untreated underactive thyroid, your risk of developing cardiovascular disease is increased.

This is because having low levels of the hormone thyroxine can lead to increased levels of cholesterol in your blood. High cholesterol can cause fatty deposits to build up in your arteries, restricting the flow of blood.

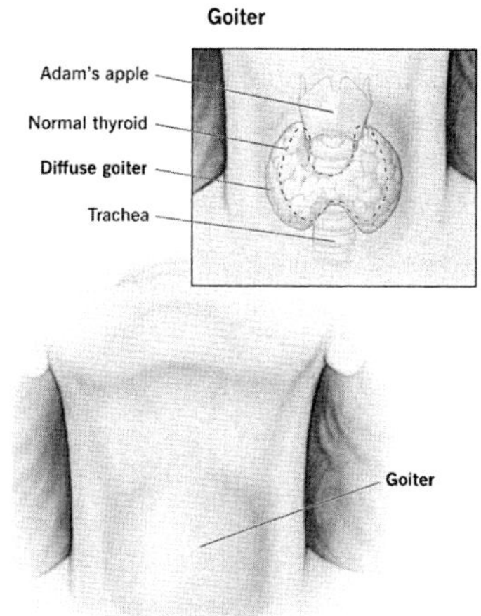

Goiter

A Goiter is an abnormal swelling of the thyroid gland, which appears as a lump in the lower neck (below the throat). Goiter can develop in people with an underactive thyroid when the body tries to stimulate the thyroid to produce more thyroid hormones.

Myxoedema coma

In very rare cases, a severe underactive thyroid may lead to a life-threatening condition called myxoedema coma. This is where the thyroid hormone levels become very low, causing symptoms such as confusion, hypothermia and drowsiness.

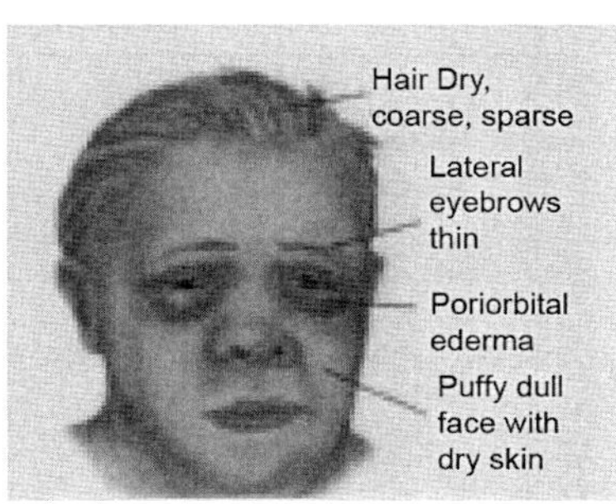

Myxoedema coma requires emergency treatment in hospital. It's usually treated with thyroid hormone replacement medicine given directly into a vein. In some cases, other treatments such as breathing support, antibiotics and steroid medicine (corticosteroids) are also required.

Complications in pregnancy

If an underactive thyroid is not treated during pregnancy, there's a risk of problems occurring. These include:

- Pre-eclampsia—which can cause high blood pressure and fluid retention in the mother and growth problems in the baby.
- Anaemia in the mother.
- An underactive thyroid in the baby.
- Birth defects/congenital deformities.
- Bleeding after child-birth.
- Problems with the baby's physical and mental development.
- Premature birth or a low birthweight baby.
- Stillbirth or miscarriage.

These problems can usually be avoided with treatment under the guidance of a specialist in hormone disorders.

Hyperthyroidism

Hyperthyroidism, also called overactive thyroid, is a condition where thyroid gland makes and releases high levels of thyroid hormone. Increase in the levels of thyroid hormone leads to increased metabolism, which leads to increased heart rate, weight loss, anxiety and behavioural changes. The main hormones of the thyroid are Triiodothyronine (T3) and Thyroxin (T4).

What causes hyperthyroidism?

1. **Graves' disease:** This disease in which thyroid makes too much thyroid hormones due to immune attack on the thyroid. It is a hereditary condition, more common in women.
2. **Thyroid nodules:** Thyroid nodule is a growth which produces more hormones than the body needs.

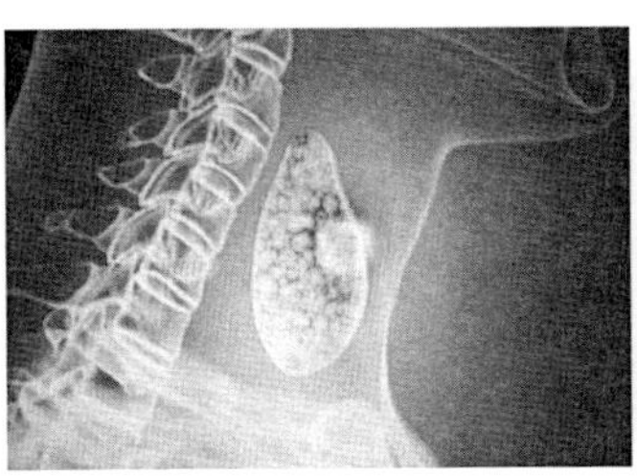

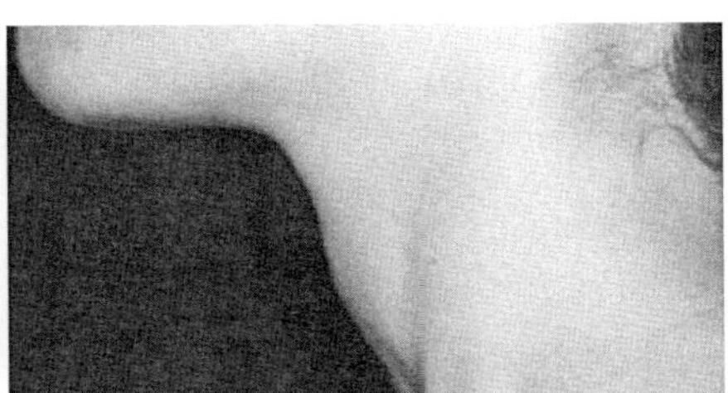

3. **Thyroiditis:** Thyroiditis is inflammation of your thyroid gland which may be painful or painless.
4. **Using excess iodine:** If people consume too much iodine through the diet or medications. Drugs used for cardiac problems called Amiodarone, which contains a high amount of iodine, can also cause hyperthyroidism.

What are the symptoms of hyperthyroidism?

- Rapid heart rate/palpitations.
- Nervousness.
- Weight loss.
- Increased appetite.
- Loose motions.
- Vision changes.
- Excessive sweating.
- Disturbed sleep.
- Hair loss.
- Bulging of the eyes.
- Muscle weakness.

What are the tests to diagnose hyperthyroidism?

- Blood test to estimate TSH, Free T3 and Free T4 levels.
- Radioactive iodine uptake (RAIU).
- Thyroid scan.
- Thyroid ultrasound.

How to treat Hyperthyroidism?

Treatment includes **anti-thyroid drugs**. Your Doctor may advise to take medicines from different groups, like

- Methimazole/carbimazole.
- Propylthiouracil (PTU).
- Radioactive iodine: radioactive iodine is an oral medicine to treat overactive thyroid.

Radioactive iodine damages these overactive thyroid cells and leads to shrinking of thyroid gland and thyroid hormones levels go down over a few weeks. This leads to permanent destruction of thyroid. Therefore, most of these patients will need Thyroid Hormone Replacement for rest of their lives.

Surgical removal of thyroid gland (Thyroidectomy) but here also the patient will need Hormone Replacement Therapy for rest of the life.

How much time after oral medications for hyperthyroidism levels start coming down?

It takes about 6-12 weeks after starting the medicines.

Can hyperthyroidism be cured?

Yes, removing thyroid gland by surgery or by destroying overactive cells by Radioactive Iodine. But then you will have to take Thyroid Hormone Replacement medicine for the rest of the life.

Thyroid Cancer

Thyroid cancer is a growth of cells that starts in the thyroid gland. Thyroid cancer may not cause any symptoms initially, but as it grows, it can cause swelling in the neck, voice changes and difficulty in swallowing.

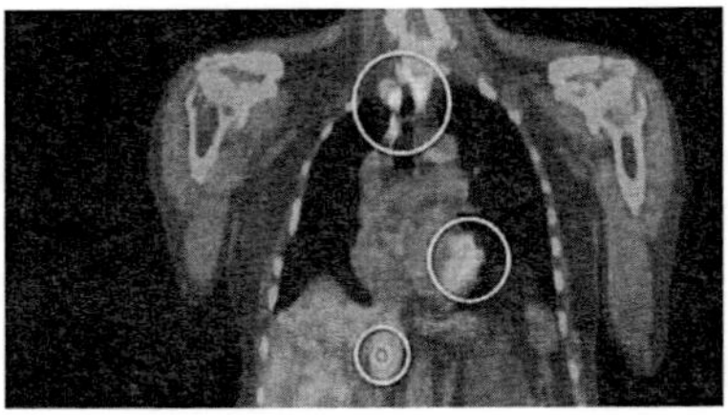

What are the symptoms of thyroid cancer?

- Swelling or growth in neck.
- Change in voice.
- Difficulty in eating/swallowing.
- Pain and discomfort in neck.
- Choking sensations in the neck.
- Weight loss.
- Tiredness.
- Loss of appetite.

Types of thyroid cancer

Papillary: 80 per cent of thyroid cancers are papillary type which grows slowly and is highly curable.

Follicular: This type of cancer is seen in 15 per cent cases of thyroid cancer. It spreads rapidly but still a curable disease in vast majority of patients.

Medullary: Medullary seen in 2 per cent of thyroid cancer. Many people with Medullary thyroid cancer may have family history of the disease.

Surgery, radioiodine therapy, hormone, radiation and chemotherapy are the options for the treatment of thyroid cancers.

Hashimoto's Thyroid

What is Hashimoto's Thyroid disease?

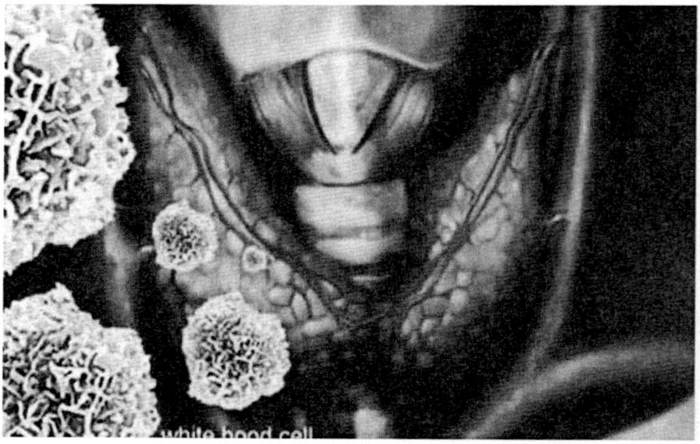

Hashimoto's disease is an autoimmune condition which causes hypothyroidism (underactive thyroid). In this condition Thyroid gland does not produce thyroid hormone. It is more commonly seen in females than in men.

Symptoms include:

- Tiredness.
- Feeling sleepy.
- Weight gain.
- Dry skin.
- Feeling cold.
- Muscle pain and joint stiffness.

- Stiffness.
- Dry brittle hair and hair loss.
- Depressed mood.
- Puffy eyes and face.
- Irregular periods.
- Infertility and decrease in sex desire.

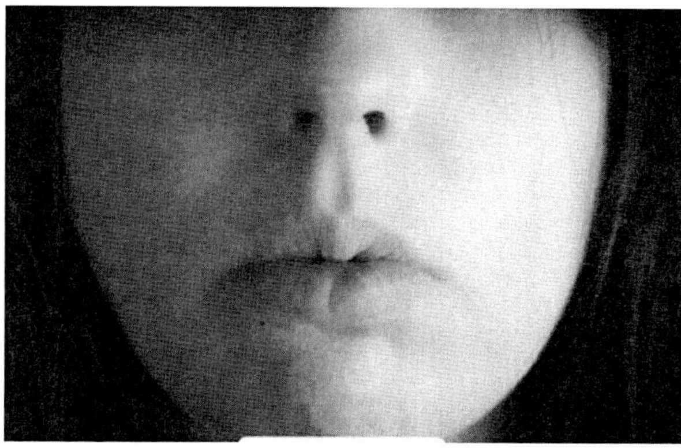

Puffy Face

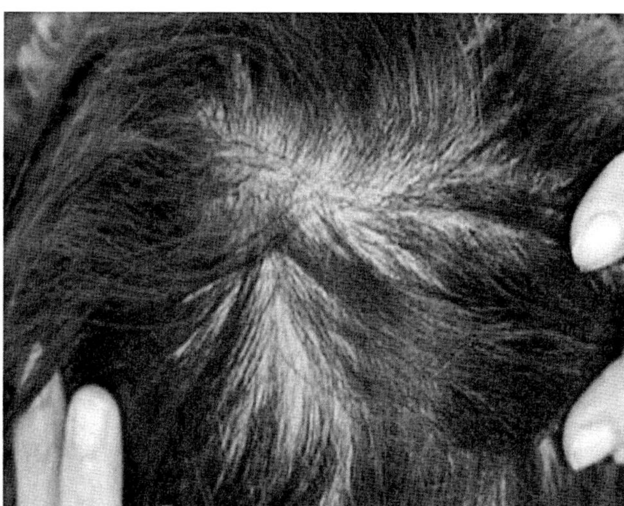

Hair Loss

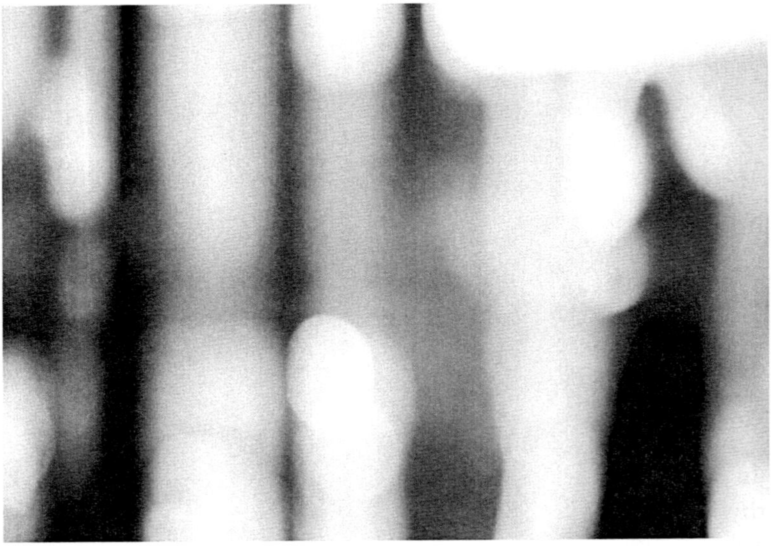

Blurred Vision

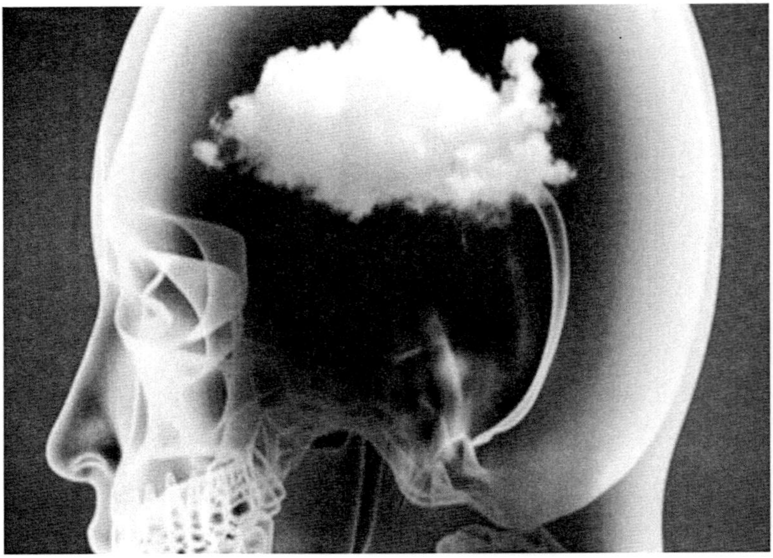

Foggy Brain

It is an autoimmune disease where antibodies attack your own thyroid tissue, which leads to less formation of thyroid hormone.

TSH levels are high and T3 and T4 levels are low.

Anti-Thyroid antibodies usually are present.

Treatment

As Hashimoto's disease leads to hypothyroidism, one needs a synthetic form of the hormone T4 called LEVOTHYROXINE. This medicine helps restore the normal levels of thyroid hormone and it has to be taken for the rest of the life. Monitor the dose by doing regular monitoring of TSH, T3 and T4 hormones.

What is the difference between Hashimoto's and Hypothyroidism?

In Hashimoto's Disease the body makes antibodies against its own thyroid gland which causes thyroid inflammation, leading to low thyroid function (hypothyroidism).

So Hashimoto's is one of the most common cause of hypothyroidism.

But there are some patients who have Hashimoto but their Thyroid is still able to work adequately and don't have hypothyroidism.

Can Hashimoto's be cured?

Currently there is no specific medicine to treat Hashimoto's but we use Levothyroxine to treat hypothyroidism which is the end effect of Hashimoto's.

Diet for Thyroid Patients

In my experience, following a Gluten free diet may improve the inflammatory response in Hashimoto's but this is not proven in the studies.

Hypothyroidism

Optimize intake of iodine containing foods, such as eggs, fish, seafood and milk.

- Use iodized salt.
- Decrease excessive intake of soy as it effects the absorption of iodine.
- **Cruciferous vegetables** such as broccoli, cauliflower, and cabbage naturally release a compound called goitrin when they are hydrolyzed or broken down in the body. Goitrin can interfere with the synthesis of thyroid hormones. However, this is usually a concern only when coupled with an iodine deficiency.

Heating cruciferous vegetables denatures much or all this potential goitrogenic effect.

For Hyperthyroid patients

Especially initially in course of treatment we should avoid seafood and other high iodine foods but this can be liberalized down the road once the condition is controlled.

I suggest to avoid soy containing foods. Apart from above mentioned I don't see any other necessary diet restrictions.

Thyroid and Weight

Thyroid disease patients can have variations in the body weight. They may lose weight or may gain weight. It depends on whether the patient is having hyperactive thyroid or hypothyroidism. There is a relationship between obesity and thyroid function.

Obese or overweight people with a normal thyroid may have higher levels of thyroid hormones and TSH in their blood. Obesity can also lead to thyroid hormone resistance, which is characterized by higher levels of TSH and free T3.

Hypothyroidism and weight gain

Hypothyroidism can cause a decrease in metabolism, which can lead to weight gain. However, not everyone with hypothyroidism will gain weight.

Weight loss and thyroid function

Weight loss can reverse the changes in thyroid hormone levels caused by obesity.

Thyroid treatment and weight

Weight gain can occur after treatment for hyperthyroidism. The mechanism for this weight gain is not fully understood.

Relationship between hypothyroidism and weight gain

Since the Body Metabolism Rate (BMR) in a person with

hypothyroidism is decreased, an underactive thyroid is generally associated with some weight gain. The weight gain is often greater in those individuals with more severe hypothyroidism. The cause of the weight gain in a hypothyroid person is also complex, and not always related to excess fat accumulation. Most of the extra weight gained in hypothyroid individuals is due to excess accumulation of salt and water. Massive weight gain is rarely associated with hypothyroidism. In general, 5-10 pounds of body weight may be attributable to the thyroid depending on the severity of the hypothyroidism.

Finally, if weight gain is the only symptom of hypothyroidism that is present, it is less likely that the weight gain is solely due to the thyroid, other symptoms of hypothyroidism like laziness, constipation and cold intolerance also be there for its diagnosis.

Once the hypothyroidism is treated, this weight gain is reversed. Since much of the weight gain in hypothyroidism is accumulation in salt and water. However, hypothyroidism usually develops over a long period of time, it is fairly common to find that there may not be any significant weight loss.

Thyroid and Diabetes

Diabetes and Thyroid disease are closely linked. If you have hyperthyroidism, your insulin levels can drop and your blood sugar can rise, increasing the risk of diabetes. If you have hypothyroidism, the opposite can occur and lead to episodes of low blood sugar.

On the other hand, Type 1 diabetes (an autoimmune form of diabetes) can increase the risk of **Hashimoto's thyroiditis** and **Graves' disease** (autoimmune forms of thyroid disease). Problems with the group of organs that produce the stress hormone cortisol, can also have a negative effect on insulin and thyroid hormone levels.

Thyroid Disease and Blood Sugar

The thyroid gland plays a major role in regulating many of our body's functions, including metabolism.

Because thyroid disease interferes with metabolism, blood sugar (glucose) that would otherwise be used for energy can instead start to accumulate. This increases the risk of diabetes, and it makes it harder to manage your blood sugar if you already have diabetes.

Hyperthyroidism (overactive thyroid) is closely linked with hyperglycemia (high blood sugar).

Hyperglycemia caused by thyroid disease can also contribute to metabolic syndrome. Metabolic syndrome is a cluster of five conditions—high glucose, high blood pressure, high triglycerides, low HDL cholesterol, and a large waist-line that increases the risk of heart disease, diabetes, and stroke.

Untreated metabolic syndrome can progress to Type 2 diabetes.

Thyroid Disease and Insulin

Thyroid disease can also interfere with the production of insulin. Insulin makes it possible for cells to use glucose for energy. This lowers blood sugar.

- Hyperthyroidism can contribute to **insulin resistance**. When you become resistant to insulin, your cells are not able to use the glucose in your blood. As a result, blood glucose levels remain high. People with diabetes who need insulin shots may also find themselves needing higher doses.
- On the other hand, hypothyroidism (an underactive thyroid) decreases metabolism. When this happens, insulin can linger, causing blood sugar to drop (hypoglycemia). For people on diabetes medications, the drop can sometimes be extreme, leading to dizziness, disorientation, and unconsciousness.

Prevention and Management

If you have been diagnosed with either thyroid disease or diabetes, achieving and maintaining your ideal weight is one of the best ways to prevent the other condition.

- Keeping your blood sugar or thyroid hormones under control can also help.
- If you have insulin resistance, in which the body does not respond to insulin as it should, thyroid disease can make your blood sugar harder to control. By managing insulin resistance with medication, diet, and exercise, you may be able to avoid diabetes as well as the complications of thyroid disease by managing hyperthyroidism with medications, diet, and exercise, you may also reduce your risk of Type 2 diabetes.

Heart Diseases Caused by Thyroid

Thyroid disorders can cause heart problems depending upon the levels of thyroid hormones.

Too much or too little of these thyroid hormones can affect the heart in different ways.

If you have an underactive thyroid, and it is not well controlled, it can make you more prone to heart problems. Or, if you already have a heart condition, it may make it worse.

Hypothyroidism or underactive thyroid can lead to

- **Slow heart rate**—Your heart rate may be slower than usual with an underactive thyroid.
- **Raise your blood pressure**—An underactive thyroid can cause arteries to stiffen, causing a rise in blood pressure. This typically affects diastolic blood pressure more than systolic blood pressure.
- **High Blood Pressure (hypertension)** increases your risk of conditions like stroke and heart attacks.
- **Increase in cholesterol levels**—One of the essential roles of thyroid hormones is to help the liver in removing excess bad cholesterol from the blood.
  Without enough T3, your levels of bad cholesterol can increase.
- **Increase your risk of coronary heart disease**—As a result of raised cholesterol, an underactive thyroid can increase your

risk of coronary heart disease. This is when your heart's blood supply is interrupted by a build-up of cholesterol and fatty substances in the artery walls called as plaque.

- People with hypothyroidism are more at risk of a **fatal cardiac event** than someone who has normal thyroid function.

Always get thyroid hormone monitoring to prevent these cardiac events.

Hyperthyroidism or overactive thyroid can lead to

- **Increased heart rate**—Your heart rate may be higher than usual and perhaps more than 100 beats per minute (known as tachycardia).
- **Raise your blood pressure**—Typically, an overactive thyroid affects systolic blood pressure more than diastolic blood pressure. This can put increased strain on the heart.
- **Palpitations**—Palpitations are noticeable rapid, strong, or irregular heartbeats. They may indicate symptom of some underlying heart rhythm/disease.
- **Trigger abnormal heart rhythms**—People with an hyperactive thyroid are more likely to develop irregular heart rate called atrial fibrillation (AF). AF is an irregular and often abnormally fast heart rate that increases the risk of blood clots in the heart. The risk of atrial fibrillation increases with age and underlying coronary heart disease.
- **Constant rapid heart rate can lead to heart failure if not treated**—An increased heart rate and blood pressure, as well as possible rhythm disturbances, can put more strain on the heart over time. Ultimately, it may lead to heart failure. This is not so common now.

Thyroid and Skin Problems

Thyroid hormone has many roles in body metabolism. These include the initiation and maintenance of hair growth, determination of epidermal thickness, and secretion of sebum.

When the amount of thyroid is excessive or reduced from normal, as may occur due to overactivity and underactivity of the thyroid gland, it may result in cutaneous changes, of various types. These skin alterations depend on the type of thyroid disease that occurs.

Hypothyroidism

The skin problems caused due to hypothyroidism are:

- **Myxedema:** This is caused by an elevated level of mucopolysaccharides (chondroitin sulfate and hyaluronic acid). These accumulate in the dermis, most prominently around the hair follicles and dermal vessels. In addition to separating the collagen bundles, they may produce some collagen degeneration.
- **Cold extremities:** A reduced core temperature and diminished skin perfusion occur due to cutaneous vasoconstriction.
- **Extremely dry skin:** This can result from decreased eccrine gland secretion. In very severe cases sweating processes may be disrupted. This results in the palms and soles becoming thick and dry, a condition known as keratoderma.

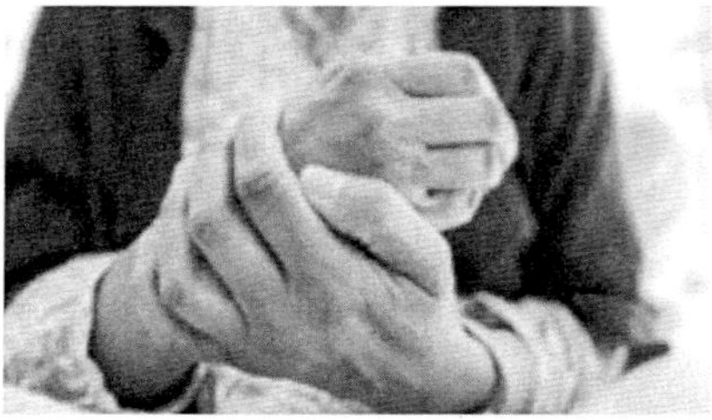

- **Carotenemia:** This refers to a yellowish discoloration on the palms and soles caused by an increased level of dermal carotene.
- **Slow growing dry, brittle, coarse hair and diminished body hair:** The drying and coarseness are considered to be partly due to the reduced secretion of sebum.
- **Madarosis:** This refers to the loss of the lateral third of the eyebrows.
- Nails are coarse, thin, and brittle and grow slowly.
- **Poor wound healing tendency:** Healing becomes slow in proportion to the degree of thyroid hormone deficiency.
- **Hypohidrosis**: This refers to an abnormal lack of sweating.
- **Xerosis:** In 57-59 per cent of patients there is a change in skin texture and poor skin hydration. This results in the skin becoming rough and covered in fine scales.

Hyperthyroidism

- **Smooth, soft, thin, warm, and moist skin:** The epidermis is thin, and the outermost skin layer is adequately hydrated.
- An increase in cutaneous blood flow causes the warmth which often occurs along with redness of the face, elbows, and palms (palmar erythema).
- **Fine, soft hair:** A diffuse non-scarring form of hair loss can also occur (**alopecia**).
- **Plummer's nails:** This is characterized by a concave contouring which raises the nails away from the nail bed.
- **Telangiectasia:** This pattern of small visible capillary vessels in a linear fashion results from breakage of capillaries in the skin.

- **Hyperhydrosis**: This abnormally excessive sweating may be observed particularly on the palms and soles.
- **Tender, red-brown nodules** occur on areas such as the shins, calves and feet.

The development of **early greying of hair**, coupled with a decrease in pigment content of hair, may present as an early symptom.

Thyroid and Eye Disease

Thyroid eye disease (TED) is an eye disorder that causes inflammation (swelling) and damage to the tissues around the eye, including muscles, fatty tissue and connective tissue. TED is an autoimmune condition, or one that happens because your protective immune system attacks your own body.

There are two phases of TED

- The active or inflammatory phase.
- The stable phase.

The active phase can last for months up to three years, while the stable phase follows when the inflammation stops.

TED is seen in some patients with Graves' disease. One out of four, approximately 25 per cent of patients in Graves' disease will develop eye disease. Rarely it can occur in absence of Graves' disease.

Whom does thyroid eye disease affect?

Thyroid eye disease happens more often in **women**. The median age for being diagnosed with TED is 43 years old. However, you can be diagnosed much earlier or much later than 43.

You may be more likely to develop thyroid eye disease if you:

- Have high levels of Thyroid antibody levels.

- Have low levels of the mineral selenium in your blood.
- Smoking or exposure to second hand smoke.

What are the signs and symptoms of thyroid eye disease?

The signs and symptoms of thyroid eye disease include:

- Dry eyes.
- Irritation in the eyes due to a gritty feeling.
- Watery eyes.
- Red eyes.
- Bulging eyes, also called proptosis.
- Double vision, also called diplopia.
- Difficulty in closing your eyes completely. This can lead to an ulcer (sore) on your cornea.
- Pain behind your eyes and pain with eye movements.

Symptoms normally affect both eyes, but sometimes you may only notice symptoms in one eye.

Is thyroid eye disease contagious?

No. Thyroid eye disease is not contagious. You can not catch it from anyone, and you cannot transmit it to anyone.

Diagnosis and Tests

What tests will be done to diagnose thyroid eye disease?

An eye doctor will be able to diagnose thyroid eye disease by doing a physical eye examination. They will be able to examine both your eyelids and your eyes.

If the eye doctor thinks that you have thyroid eye disease, they will order blood tests to check if your thyroid hormone levels and if the antibodies are too high or too low.

Other tests your health-care provider may request include:

- Ultrasound of the eyes.
- Computed tomography (CT SCAN) of the eyes.
- Magnetic resonance imaging (MRI) of the eyes.

Lifestyle changes and home remedies to treat TED

The most important lifestyle change you can make is to quit smoking if you smoke. It raises your risk of developing TED by seven to eight times and makes TED's active (inflammatory) disease phase longer. In addition, smoking decreases the effectiveness of treatment for thyroid eye disease. Other things you can do to be more comfortable include:

- Using cool compresses on your eyes.
- Wearing sunglasses.
- Keeping your head higher than your body when you lie down.
- Taping your eyelids shut when you sleep. (Being unable to close your eyes can lead to dryness and a corneal ulcer, which can cause scars on your eyes and loss of vision.)
- Wearing glasses with prisms to reduce double vision.
- Using a patch on one eye to reduce double vision.

Keep your thyroid hormone level near normal by following your doctors suggestions and getting regular thyroid tests done.

Surgery to treat TED

Eyelid surgery: Tight eyelids keep your top eyelid from coming down and your bottom lid from coming up. This can lead to corneal damage. Eyelid surgery may make it easier to keep your cornea covered.

Eye muscle surgery: Your provider may recommend surgery to move your eye muscles and help to correct double vision. You may need more than one surgery.

Orbital decompression surgery: This surgery relieves the pressure on the optic nerve by making the eye socket larger or taking away excess tissue. The surgery lessens the burden of the eye. If your provider recommends other surgeries (eyelid, eye muscle), orbital decompression is usually done first.

Thyroid and Pregnancy

Thyroid hormones are crucial for normal development of your baby's brain and nervous system.

- During the first trimester (the first 3 months of pregnancy—baby depends on the mother for supply of thyroid hormone, which comes through the placenta).
- At around 12 weeks, your baby's thyroid starts to work on its own, but it doesn't make enough thyroid hormone until 18 to 20 weeks of pregnancy.
- Two pregnancy-related hormones—human chorionic gonadotropin (hCG) and estrogen—cause higher levels of thyroid hormone in the blood.

Thyroid problems can be hard to diagnose in pregnancy due to higher levels of thyroid hormones and other symptoms that occur in both pregnancy and thyroid disorders.

Hyperthyroidism in Pregnancy

Some signs and symptoms of hyperthyroidism often occur in normal pregnancies, including:

- Faster heart rate.
- Heat intolerance and tiredness.
- Fast and irregular heartbeat.
- Shaky hands/tremors in hand.

- Unexplained weight loss or failure to have normal pregnancy weight gain.

What causes hyperthyroidism in pregnancy?

Hyperthyroidism in pregnancy is usually caused by **Graves' disease**. Graves' disease is an autoimmune disorder. With this disease, your immune system makes antibodies that cause the thyroid to make too much thyroid hormones. This antibody is called thyroid stimulating immunoglobulin or TSI.

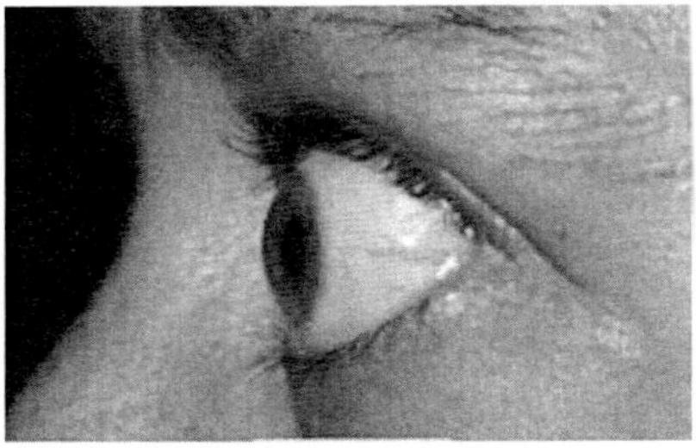

- Graves' disease may first appear during pregnancy. However, if you already have Graves' disease, your symptoms could improve in your second and third trimesters.
- Your immune system is less active later in pregnancy so the immune system makes less TSI, so the symptoms improve.
- Graves' disease often gets worse again in the first few months after the baby is born, when TSI levels go up again.

Thyroid hormone levels that are too high can harm the health of the mother and the baby.

How can hyperthyroidism affect the pregnancy?

Untreated hyperthyroidism during pregnancy can lead to

- Miscarriage.
- Premature birth.
- Low birthweight.
- Pre-eclampsia—A dangerous rise in blood pressure in late pregnancy.

- Thyroid storm—A sudden, severe worsening of symptoms.
- Congestive heart failure.
- Rarely, Graves' disease may also affect a baby's thyroid, causing it to make too much thyroid hormone.

Even if your hyperthyroidism was cured by radioactive iodine treatment to destroy thyroid cells or surgery to remove your thyroid, your body still makes the TSI antibody. When levels of this antibody are high, TSI may travel to your baby's bloodstream. Just as TSI caused your own thyroid to make too much thyroid hormone, it can also cause your baby's thyroid to make too much of thyroid hormone.

What are the symptoms of hypothyroidism in pregnancy?

Symptoms of an underactive thyroid are often the same for pregnant women as for other people with hypothyroidism. Symptoms include:

- Extreme tiredness,
- Increased sensitivity to cold.
- Muscle cramps,
- Severe constipation, and
- Problems with memory or concentration.

What causes hypothyroidism in pregnancy?

Hypothyroidism in pregnancy is usually caused by **Hashimoto's disease**. Hashimoto's disease is an autoimmune disorder. In Hashimoto's disease, the immune system makes antibodies that attack the thyroid, causing inflammation and damage that make it less able to make thyroid hormones.

How can hypothyroidism affect the mother and baby?

Untreated hypothyroidism during pregnancy can lead to—

- Pre-eclampsia—a dangerous rise in blood pressure in late pregnancy.
- Anaemia.

- Miscarriage.
- Low birthweight.
- Stillbirth.
- Congestive heart failure, rarely.

These problems occur most often with severe hypothyroidism. Because thyroid hormones are so important to the baby's brain and nervous system development, untreated hypothyroidism—especially during the first trimester—can cause low IQ and problems with normal development of the baby.

If you are on medicines for hypothyroidism, then during pregnancy the dose has to be readjusted.

Thyroid and Infertility

How can Thyroid Disorders affect your fertility?

Hypothyroidism and hyperthyroidism can each negatively impact fertility—both the ability to become pregnant and the ability to carry a fetus to term. The presence of autoimmune antibodies, with or without hyper or hypothyroidism, can also impact your fertility.

Abnormal TSH levels can interfere with ovulation, and when you have any type of thyroid disorder (without proper management), you will see a luteal phase (the last half of the cycle after ovulation) disruption.

This is mediated by progesterone levels. If a thyroid disorder is unregulated, a patient could have difficulty getting pregnant because there will not be implantation. One could also experience early miscarriage because of incomplete implantation in the uterine wall.

Signs of low levels or misfunctioning of progesterone

- A shorter or longer cycle than your typical menstrual cycle.
- Lighter or heavier bleeding than is typical for you.

Fertility is not a female-only concern. Thyroid disorders in men can also affect a couple's fertility. Dysregulated thyroid function can damage sperm quality and motility, making it difficult for the sperm to enter the egg for fertilization.

Lifestyle Interventions

- Vitamin D can also play a role in keeping your thyroid healthy. Some recent studies show promising results that Vitamin D may also help to lower thyroid antibodies. Vitamin D is easy to find in supplement form (if you are not getting enough from the sun).
- Selenium is another important nutrient for thyroid health. Brazil nuts are an excellent source.

Thyroid and Sexual Dysfunction

Sexual intimacy is an integral part of a relationship. Sexual dysfunction or the lack of desire for sex can cause rifts and other problems in family life. It affects not only the relationship but also a person's physical self-esteem. Further, it may be an indicator of other severe health problems such as thyroid.

Thyroid hormones control the way your body uses energy. If your levels of thyroid hormone are low, many of your body processes can slow down. This may lead to a loss of sex drive.

Common hypothyroidism symptoms like fatigue and weight gain may also impact your desire for sex. Hypothyroidism may cause elevated levels of the hormone prolactin.

Effects of thyroid on the sexual life

Hypothyroidism symptoms such as weight gain, irregular or heavier than usual menstrual periods and thinning hair can often be embarrassing and uncomfortable for people with the condition to deal with. Another potentially embarrassing symptom, however, often goes unreported—sexual dysfunction or a weakening libido.

It is extremely common for women with an underactive thyroid to have some sort of sexual dysfunction.

Painful Sex

Higher-than-normal levels of this hormone can contribute to vaginal dryness.The dry vaginal skin is a symptom of thyroid disease in women. Vaginal dryness will make sexual intercourse unpleasant, resulting in a decreased desire for sexual activity.

Decreased testosterone

It is possible to have low testosterone if you suffer from a thyroid disorder. Thyroid disorders can also lower your libido. Although testosterone is considered a "man's hormone", it is produced by both men and women. Both men and women rely on it for different levels of sex drive.

Ejaculation disorders

Men with thyroid issues may experience ejaculation problems, whether its premature or delayed. These issues may be a result of thyroid issues. Hypothyroidism increases the chance of delayed ejaculation, and hyperthyroidism increases the chance of premature ejaculation, according to the Sexual Medicine Society of North America (SMSNA).

Erectile dysfunction

Hormonal imbalances caused by thyroid disorders may make it challenging for men to get or keep an erection. The condition is relatively common, especially among hypothyroid men.

The prevalence of sexual dysfunction in patients with hypothyroid (59-63% and 22-46% in men and women, respectively) and hyperthyroidism (48-77% and 44-60% in men and women, respectively) has been estimated in select populations as per studies. The major problems include lack of vaginal lubrication, decreased libido and Erectile Dysfunction (ED).

FAQs

Does only women have thyroid issues?

Thyroid diseases occur more commonly in women than men, because of the autoimmune nature of many thyroid disorders. Hypothyroidism, and thyroid nodules occur frequently in both pre- and post-menopausal women. Pregnancy is also associated with changes in thyroid functions.

Are thyroid problems always hereditary?

Researchers have discovered gene variants (mutations) associated with thyroid disease and suggest that up to 65 per cent of thyroid hormone production is determined by genetics, indicating that a family history increases the risk.

Do all thyroid patients gain weight?

Since the BMR in the patient with hypothyroidism is decreased, an underactive thyroid is generally associated with some weight gain. The weight gain is often greater in those individuals with severe hypothyroidism.

Weight gain may signal low levels of thyroid hormones, a condition called hypothyroidism. In contrast, if the thyroid produces more hormones than the body needs, you may lose weight unexpectedly. This is seen in hyperthyroidism.

Is TSH a good indicator of thyroid function?

Occasionally, a low TSH may result from an abnormality in the pituitary gland, which prevents it from making enough TSH to stimulate the thyroid (central hypothyroidism). In most healthy individuals, a normal TSH value means that the thyroid is functioning properly.

Is hypothyroidism the only thyroid disorder?

The two main types of thyroid disease are hypothyroidism and hyperthyroidism. Both conditions can be caused by other diseases that impact the way the thyroid gland works. Conditions that can cause hypothyroidism include:

Thyroiditis: This condition is an inflammation (swelling) of the thyroid gland.

One can't manage thyroid health through lifestyle changes.

Managing the thyroid can be difficult, but by following a healthy and active lifestyle one can maintain this easily. Take medications as prescribed by your doctor, eat a healthy diet, practice yoga, exercise daily, and practice stress-reducing exercises like deep breathing to manage your thyroid health.

Are thyroid disorders always accompanied by obvious symptoms

Thyroid gland problems tend to develop slowly, often over several years. At first, one may barely notice the symptoms of hypothyroidism, such as fatigue and weight gain. Or you may think they are just part of getting older. But as your metabolism continues to slow, you may develop more obvious problems.

Do's and Don'ts in Thyroid

Do's

1. ***Check thyroid regularly***

It is important to check thyroid levels regularly—by testing TSH levels empty stomach early in the morning. At times, a doctor may completely depend upon the blood test for diagnosis and overlook thyroid dysfunction. This may leave many people undiagnosed. Therefore, it is important to have a clear discussion with your doctor about your symptoms and seek clarity.

2. ***Maintain good hydration***

3. ***Eat selenium, tyrosine, and antioxidants rich food***

Seafood, nuts, fruits, brazil nuts, kidney and liver contain Selenium—an enzyme that converts T4 to T3, Tyrosine-based food includes almonds, sesame seeds, oats etc. Antioxidants rich food includes all fresh vegetables and fruits. These foods will reduce inflammation and help enhance health.

Don'ts

1. ***Avoid smoking or drinking alcohol***

Thyroid patients, if they smoke or drink alcohol, should put a stop to these immediately. This is because alcohol is a depressant and it suppresses the thyroid gland functions. Tobacco or smoking is equally harmful as it blocks the synthesis of hormones.

2. *Stay away from sugar and caffeine*

Caffeine tends to stress the body and so does sugar. Consuming caffeine in smaller quantities is good as it helps to manage inflammation, by opening up the blood vessels. However, consuming more than the recommended amount of caffeine can alter the TSH levels produced by the pituitary glands.

4. *No self-medication*

Most often thyroid patients struggle to understand what's happening to their body and therefore, they turn to the internet for reference. The internet with its wide range of sources tells different stories and patients get carried away and start to relate everything happening in their body to be a thyroid problem.

Nutritional Therapy in Thyroid

Medical nutritional therapy in Hypothyroidism

What to Eat	What Not to Eat
• Whole eggs, fish, crab, lobster, mollusks, sardines, salmon, organ meats such as liver, muscle meat. • Milk and dairy products—milk, cheese, yogurt etc. • Grains and brazil nuts. Dried beans, lentils, and other legumes. • Nuts, including pine nuts, walnuts, almonds, and pistachios. • Vegan sources: fortified cereals and nutritional yeast.	• Fast-food meals. • Salty processed foods, sugary treats such as pastry, cake, cookies, and ice cream. • Excessive alcohol and soy-based foods. • Cruciferous vegetable, viz. broccoli, cabbage, brussels sprouts, cauliflower and kale. • Turnips and gluten containing foods: Bread, pasta, millets.

Medical nutritional therapy in Hyperthyroidism

What to Eat	What Not to Eat
• Non-Iodized Salt. • Egg Whites. • Fresh or Canned Fruits. • Nuts, Breads, Dairy Oats, Potatos, Honey, Bamboo Shoots, Seeds and Whole Grains, Mushrooms, Chickpeas and Meat. • Green Leafy Vegetables, Broccoli, Brussels Sprouts, Cauliflower, Kale, Mustard, Spinach, White Beans and Okra. Dried Beans, Lentils, Poultry, and Red Meat.	• Beverages Like Coffee and Tea. • Certain Fruits: Peaches, Pears and Strawberries. • Fish, Seaweed and Sushi. • Cheese, Egg Yolk, Iodized Salt. • Soy Milk, Soy Sauce and Soy-based Creamers.

Goitrogens

- Cruciferous vegetables such as broccoli, cauliflower, and cabbage naturally release a compound called goitrin when they are hydrolyzed or broken down. Goitrin can interfere with the synthesis of thyroid hormones. However, this is usually a concern only when coupled with an iodine deficiency. Heating cruciferous vegetables denatures much or all this potential goitrogenic effect.
- Soy is another potential goitrogen. It can interrupt absorption of thyroid drugs so that patients with subclinical hypothyroidism are prone to develop hypothyroidism. The isoflavones in soy can lower Thyroid Hormone Synthesis.
- The potential exception is millet, a nutritious gluten-free grain, which may suppress thyroid function even in people with adequate iodine intake. If a dietary recall indicates frequent millet consumption in patients with hypothyroidism, it may be wise to suggest they choose a different grain.
- Flavonoids: in fruits, vegetables, and tea have antioxidant properties and cardiovascular benefits. However, the high levels of flavonoid supplements may suppress the thyroid function. They interfere with the metabolism of TSH by reducing the T4 levels in serum and inhibiting both the conversion of T4 to T3, flavonoid with antioxidant potential reduces thyroid peroxidase, the enzyme responsible for the oxidation of iodide and formation of thyroid hormones, T3 and T4 levels with a concomitant raise of TSH.